RECIPE FOR TRUE FITNESS

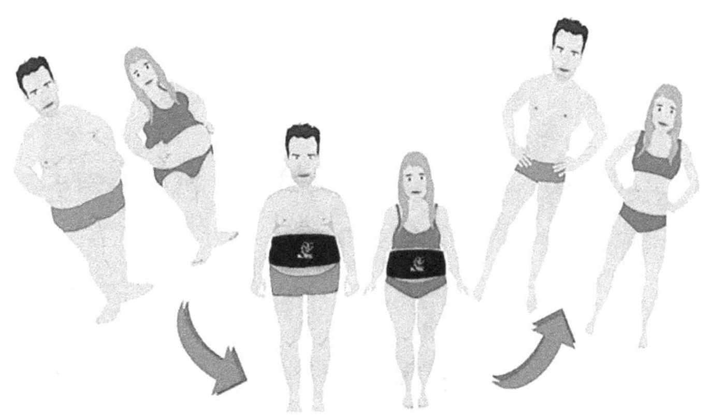

Written By MJ West Solutions

Disclaimer: MJ West Solutions provides health and fitness suggestions that are designed to improve quality of life. Always consult a physician before starting a new exercise program or diet.

ISBN: 978-1-64316-505-9

Table of Contents

Introduction

What is true fitness?

Would you like to know what it really means to be Truly Fit? Well, I will go straight to the point, and I am sure you will be surprised.

True Fitness is a lifestyle. It's about having a certain mindset, a certain attitude towards yourself. Yes, it's about having the body and health you want, but it's first and foremost about loving yourself deeply from the inside. It's about knowing who you really are. True fitness is about growing mentally, physically and spiritually; it's not something that comes quickly. It's the result of a complete transformation of your inner being and the sum of daily positive and healthy habits.

The three main ways of attaining true fitness are engaging in physical activities, healthy nutrition and getting enough sleep.

Fitness equals working on the internal aspects and external aspects of yourself. Usually, you only think about the external aspects. But you have to first become the person inside that you desire to reflect on the outside. That's why it's better that you work on the inside part (nutrition and sleep) and the outside part (physical activity). This will help you achieve true fitness in no time.

To help you on your way, in this e-book, I'll be sharing with you the roles that sleep, nutrition, and physical activity play in true fitness. First, let›s talk about habits: You will not reach fitness in one day, and the new lifestyle it requires will not come in one minute either. You have to install new positive habits each day. You have to be mentally prepared, and this takes some time and work! Once you are truly committed to fitness, you will experience three phases you must master:

One is the **motivation phase**, where you will be super charged with energy and happy to undertake what you decided to. This phase is usually the easiest one. The second phase is the **discipline phase**, where your motivation starts to fade away. This is the most critical part. Your body hasn't yet accepted the new habits, so it tries to keep you away from going forward. In this phase, you must be disciplined and not listen to your negative or restraining feelings.

You must hold onto your vision, as you've not yet seen the results you are seeking. Just control your mind and keep going, whatever your thoughts are. The third phase is the **rewarding phase**. Here you start seeing your first results... and your motivation comes back! It's a sign your body has accepted your new programming. Your feelings are now positive and you enjoy your new state of being.

It's all about patience and having strong faith in what you're doing and why you've undertaken what you envision. New habits don't come quickly, but think about the rewards they bring! One key factor to stay motivated and to manifest what you truly desire is to strongly believe in yourself and your potential. You can make it! Practice daily positive affirmations, imagining yourself in the new situation and enjoying this future state (i.e., feeling healthy, full of energy, having a beautiful body, etc.).

Why people fail to gain true fitness

Many people only look for the quick fix and fail to recognize that true fitness involves the entire human element—the body, mind and spirit. Statistics will reveal that those who've adopted the fitness lifestyle are able to deal with the daily stresses of life, maintain good physical and mental health, and actually want to continue proper sleeping, nutrition and exercise habits.

How important is your exercise routine and the overall health of your body? Participating in physical activities teaches the body to work as a cohesive unit and allows one to understand how each body part affects another. People who have developed the abilities to survive and flourish in their natural environments, through genetics or proper training, tend to develop the hard, lean, and muscular bodies that many strive for.

In this e-book, I'll be showing you the roles that physical activity, nutrition, and sleep play in true fitness. Just remember: Physical activity, good diet, and good sleep every day are the keys to true fitness.

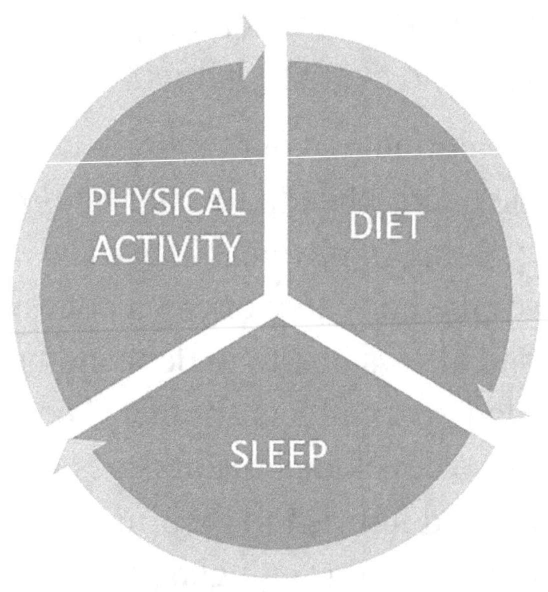

TRUE FITNESS

How Physical Activity, Nutrition, and Sleep Helps You Attain True Fitness

They help you control weight

Engaging in physical activities, getting enough sleep, and watching your diet can help prevent excess weight gain or help maintain weight loss. When you are engaged in physical activity, you burn calories. The more intense the activity, the more calories you burn.

Regular trips to the gym are great, but don't worry if you can't find a large chunk of time to exercise every day. To reap the benefits of exercise, just get more active throughout your day—take the stairs instead of the elevator or rev up your household chores. Consistency is key.

They help combat health conditions and diseases

Worried about heart disease? Hoping to prevent high blood pressure? No matter what your current weight, being active boosts high-density lipoprotein (HDL), or "good" cholesterol, and decreases unhealthy triglycerides. This one-two punch keeps your blood flowing smoothly, which decreases your risk of cardiovascular diseases.

Physical activity, good sleep, and good diet helps you stay fit, and also prevent or manage a wide range of health problems and concerns, including stroke, metabolic syndrome, type 2 diabetes, depression, a number of types of cancer, arthritis, and falls.

They help boost your energy

Doing these things regularly can improve your muscle strength and boost your endurance.

They help in delivering oxygen and nutrients to your tissues and help your cardiovascular system work more efficiently. When your heart and lung health improve, you have more energy and fitness.

Physical activity and nutrition promote better sleep

Struggling to snooze? Regular physical activity and good diet can help you fall asleep faster and deepen your sleep. Just don't exercise or eat too close to bedtime, or you may be too energized to hit the hay. Now you can see how the three are connected in helping you gain true fitness.

They give you more vim and vigor

Doing these things are like taking nature's energy drink, firing up your brain and body so you feel more alert and alive. Engaging in physical activities, eating good meals, and getting enough rest puts your body in a state of arousal, which translates into more vitality and a greater sense of wellbeing. Daily tasks become less strenuous and require less exertion.

They help improve your blood flow

As you age, it's not only joints that can get stiff—the blood vessels in your body can lose their flexibility. This makes it harder for them to expand and contract as needed to deliver oxygen-rich blood to parts of the body that need it the most (like the brain, heart, and muscles). And stiffer arteries can raise your blood pressure, meaning your heart has to work harder to pump blood through them. Doing these things daily can lower blood pressure, improve circulation, and ensure you reach true fitness.

The Power of Fruits, Vegetables, and Spices

Fruits are a major component of a balanced and healthy eating plan; they are a vital source of minerals, vitamins, and fibers that are required for good health. Fruit with high contents of fiber and pectin work as a fat burner and can also enhance the metabolic system; there are several fruits that are low in fat and calories. What's more, many of these fruits are packed with antioxidants (1). They include:

Avocado

Avocado contains omega-9 fatty acids, which is the type of fatty acids existing in macadamia nuts and olives. The omega-9 fatty acid can improve fat metabolism, break down fat rapidly, and prevent excessive fat accumulation in the system (2, 3).

Coconut

Coconuts are rich in medium chain fatty acids (MCFAs); this compound has been associated with reducing cholesterol capacity in the liver and other tissues. MCFAs are also found in coconut derivatives such as coconut flour and shredded (unsweetened) coconut while coconut oil has been reported to aid thyroid gland functioning (4, 5). Coconut is also a type of fruit that can fill the belly and prevent the urge to consume unhealthy snacks.

Lemons

This fruit enhances the detoxification reactions of the liver while maintaining the alkaline content of the body. The impact of lemon on liver health is crucial to the digestion process, including fat metabolism and its digestion (6, 7).

Grapefruit

Scientists have been able to prove that regular consumption of grapefruit is an effective means to lose weight (8, 9). Although grapefruit does not burn fat, its high water content can make you feel full. Consequently, you will consume less calories during meals.

Tomatoes

High in lycopene, it also promotes the formation of carnitine, which has been shown to be effective in fat burning.

Other recommended fruit includes watermelons, blueberries, apples, pears, and bananas.

A report from the European Journal of Clinical Nutrition (2014 edition) revealed that those who consumed an increased proportion of vegetables were able to burn a significant amount of fat within 90 days. In comparison, those who reduced their consumption of vegetables received less flattering results. Vegetables are essential for diet as they play specific roles in maintaining a healthy body. Some fresh vegetables offer more nutrients than others and are more beneficial to a weight-loss plan. Green vegetables such as broccoli, baby spinach, and kale contain high quantities of phytonutrients, some of which play a significant role in fat burning. Such phytonutrient may include flavonoids and carotenoids which have potent antioxidant properties. Lettuce and cucumbers are also very valuable vegetables for this purpose. Apart from green vegetables, some other colored vegetables are also great in the fat process scheme; examples are the white cauliflower, purple eggplant, and yellow winter squash.

ORANGE AND YELLOW VEGETABLES

This class of vegetables is useful not only for burning fats but also for the eyes, heart and skin. Beta-carotene is a major phytonutrient present in this class of vegetables, which is required for proper functioning of the eyes and skin. This beta-carotene is also the precursor for vitamin A, which is designed to destroy oxidative stress. Additionally, orange and yellow vegetables are rich in Vitamin C, which helps fight belly fat and reduces stress hormones in the body. Typical examples of orange and yellow vegetables are yellow tomatoes, carrots, corn, pumpkin, summer squash, sweet potatoes, and yellow/orange peppers.

GREEN VEGETABLES

These are good sources of vitamin A and vitamin C; they also play a significant role in reducing oxidative stress, belly fat and the level of stress hormones to maintain a healthy body. The folic acid content in these vegetables enhance digestion of protein. Folic acid sees the proper metabolism of protein in the body and maintains its insulin level. Unstable insulin levels in the body can trigger fat deposit and storage in the belly. However, eating an adequate amount of vegetables rich in folic acid will help stabilize insulin levels and decrease the storage of belly fat. Examples of such vegetables are cabbage, broccoli, asparagus, Brussels sprouts, cucumbers, lettuce, kale, green beans, and zucchini.

WHITE VEGETABLES

These groups of vegetables contain anthoxanthin and allicin, which are active compounds that aid in fighting diseases. They can reduce the overall cholesterol and blood pressure level in the body. Examples include mushroom, onions, parsnips, cauliflower, and turnips.

RED AND PURPLE VEGETABLES

This class contains the lycopene, which is an antioxidant compound, and has been reported to be anti-carcinogenic. Lycopene can improve heart health, reduce high blood pressure, and promote strong bones. Examples are beets, red cabbage, eggplants, and tomatoes.

SPICES AID IN FAT LOSS

Some spices have been found to reduce belly fat (12), these include:

Ginseng

This is one of the best spices for fat loss. Commonly available ones are the Chinese ginseng and the Siberian ginseng. It is widely available as a tea or as a supplement. The primary active component of this plant is caffeine, which enhances metabolism and also helps to increase energy levels.

Turmeric

This popular spice is often used in Indian cuisine. It is essential for burning fat and losing excess weight.

Peppermint

Peppermint works by removing waste and toxins from the body. It also helps to reduce bloating and aids in digestion. Peppermint is helpful for those losing weight as it reduces stress and suppresses appetite (13).

Garlic

This enhances fat metabolism and reduces the rate at which the body stores fat.

Dandelion

This is a perfect weed for burning fat and promoting weight loss. Every part—flowers, root, and leaves—is utilized for this purpose. Dandelion neutralizes toxins in the body and helps to reduce inflammation. It can be taken as a tea, consumed as leaves in a salad, or as a supplement.

Energy-Boosting Fruits

Fruit contains vitamins, antioxidants and minerals, and fiber which can give an instant energy boost. The calorie level available in fruits differs; some fruits may contain about 80 to 120 calories.

1. Bananas

    Bananas have substantial content of easily digestible fiber, and also contain a large quantity of potassium and other electrolytes. They give an instant energy boost on consumption, and also maintain proper functioning of the nerves and muscle. One medium banana contains about 105 calories, 27 grams of carbs, 1 gram of protein and 0.5 grams of fat.

2. Papaya

    Papaya has been identified as a potential medicinal plant, and taking papaya juice has been shown to be effective in fighting the common cold and rheumatoid arthritis.

3. Oranges

    They are high energy-giving fruits with a large quantity of organic sugar and vitamin C. The natural sugar is essential in reducing fatigue and stress.

4. Strawberries

    They are energy-giving fruits required for fighting fatigue while enhancing vision. A cup of strawberries has been shown to contain about 80 mg of Vitamin C, which is significantly higher than that of oranges (70 mg).

5. Pineapple

    Pineapple is not only an energy-producing food, it also delivers manganese, copper, vitamins C, B1 and B6, and fiber.

Six Tips to Help You along Your Weight Loss Journey

Exercise early in the day, preferably within two hours of waking up. Your body is well rested and energized after 6-8 hours of quality sleep. This is the perfect time to expose yourself to a challenging workout. Morning exercise is just as important as a good breakfast. During my time as a First Sergeant in the U.S. Army, I always referred to our Physical Training as "Good Breakfast." No pancakes, eggs and sausage, just a great morning physical training session; a wholesome traditional breakfast comes afterwards.

Find a workout partner who is willing to hold you accountable for being lazy or taking shortcuts during the workout. This enables you to stay on track during periods of weakness.

Make your body pay for consumption of excess calories. The average man needs approximately 2500 calories daily while women need about 2000 calories. Studies show increased activity may require men and women to consume more calories. We should always strive to get our calories from healthy foods, but things happen. If you must consume unhealthy snacks or meals, enjoy them now and pay for them later. Find out how many calories you consumed and determine how you can burn those calories during your next workout session.

Challenge your body by exposing it to different workouts and levels of intensity. The body tends to get bored when you feed it the same workouts, and as a result, it stops reacting. Many people get frustrated after failing to achieve desired results. I learned earlier that changing up my workout would lead to better outcomes. Gradually increase resistance levels, repetitions, and energy during the workout.

Conduct oral hygiene at least three hours before bedtime. According to most dentists, it takes two to three minutes to brush your teeth. It should take the average person with 28 teeth about two minutes to floss. Lastly, rinsing with mouth wash should take about 30 seconds. It is safe to say that the average person spends at least five minutes and thirty seconds conducting oral hygiene at night. Conducting oral hygiene at least three hours before bedtime can help prevent eating close to bedtime.

After spending a significant amount of effort brushing, flossing and rinsing, I am not interested in consuming more food. In the end, I eat less and wake up in the morning feeling lighter on my feet.

Commit yourself to the idea of achieving your desired size. Purchase an expensive pair of pants, a shirt, or a skirt that reflects the size you desire to be. If you wear a size 16 and want to be a size 8, buy a size 8. Place the item in a closet area that is highly visible; this will serve as a constant reminder of your goal.

Using MJ West Solutions Waist Trimmer

When it comes to working out, people who want to lose some extra pounds have to understand that the most effective way to lose weight is through a balanced diet, good sleep and regular exercise.

Apart from this, there are a few safe supplements and add-ons to workouts which may help you to shape your body. One of these add-ons is the **MJ West Solutions Waist Trimmer Belt.**

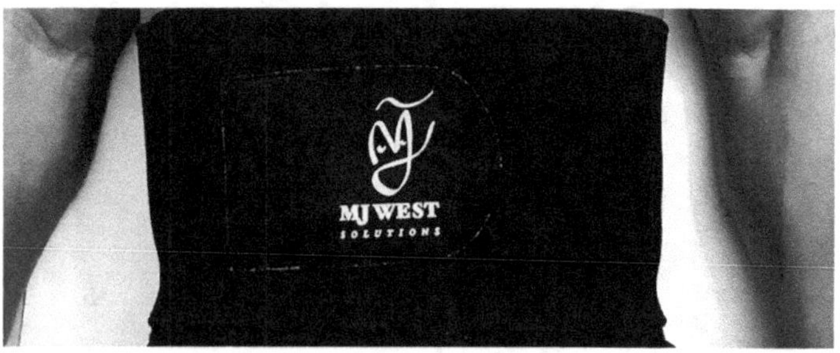

(Belt available at mjwest.solutions and amazon.com)

Your stomach is one of the areas of your body where fat gets stored, and it is also one of the most difficult places to remove the fat from.

The surplus water in your body also gets stored in your stomach, and no amount of exercise can reduce that surplus water. MJ West Solutions waist trimmer tightens around your abdominal area and helps your body to sweat out the water from the stomach area.

What is a Waist Trimmer Belt? - Waist trimmer belts help to trim your abdominal region.

It is made of thick neoprene fabric, which is comfortable, durable and lightweight. It can be worn around your waist when you perform your normal workouts. The belt retains the heat from your abdomen and helps you to sweat off water weight from this area.

Our waist trimmer belt can help reduce weight because the added heat in your midsection and lower back help you to get rid of water weight. It is very important to stay hydrated while you wear a waist trimmer belt.

Some people find this belt useful because this belt supports their back or helps reduce pain while they exercise. The waist trimmer belt is flexible enough to allow you free movement.

How Does MJ West Solutions Waist Trimmer Belt Work?

Our waist trimmer belts work by accumulating more heat from the body during exercise and retaining your body temperature.

Normally, a human body releases the heat produced during exercise, but the trimmer belts retain the heat in your body so that you can burn more calories and the excess water in your waistline can be reduced quickly.

The belts are usually worn around the midsection and provide back support as you exercise. While you work out, it is important to maintain good body posture to trim down fat quickly and to target muscles properly.

The belts also speed up your metabolism rate as they help burn calories two times faster while you do conventional workouts.

Do Waist Trimmers **Work?**

Even though the results of wearing a waist trimmer belt may vary between people, consistent use helps to shed a few pounds.

The weight loss may be due to loss of water weight and it may be temporary. The belt causes you to keep your stomach tight during a workout and this helps to tone the stomach muscles.

Some believe that a waist trimmer belt helps to eliminate more toxins because you sweat more, but you have to eat a balanced diet, get good sleep and follow a proper exercise regimen when you use waist trimmer belts to get better results.

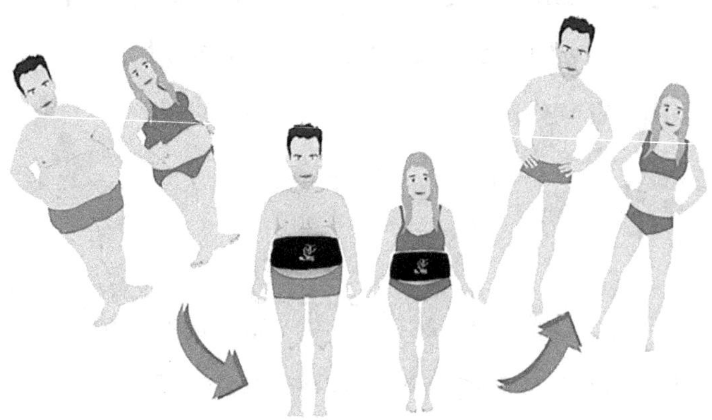

How to Use a Waist Trimmer Belt?

It is important for the waist trimmer belt to rest against your skin, so remove all upper body clothing like shirts and larger sports bras.

Wrap the trimmer belt around your waist so that the thicker part of the belt fits in your back. Stretch the belt around your stomach and wrap around the other side of the belt and fasten with the Velcro lining. You can wear your clothing over the waist trimmer belt.

Perform your usual workouts, from jogging to weightlifting. The waist trimmer belt will heat up your stomach area, which is covered with the belt, and will cause it to sweat more than usual. After completing your workout, you can remove the belt and wash it.

Our waist trimmers are destined to be a global favorite. The greatest advantage of using these waist trimmer belts is that your body has complete freedom to mobilize. Unlike those inflexible corsets and waist trainers, these belts do provide practical results, and you do not have to behave like a rigid robot.

Weight loss does not mean that you have to go out of your comfort zone and keep yourself in heaps of pain. When you are comfortable, you can wear it longer for even better results. These trimmers work to solve potential problems with weight in a precise manner. It generates heat in the midsection and gets rid of that surplus water around your belly. These belts are ideal for personal health because they not only contribute towards your weight loss regime, but also provide improved support to your back and keep your posture straight, making you look and feel great. Get your waist trimmer today and get additional support when you work out.

Conclusion

You Need To Make True Fitness Your Top Priority

Imagine what you could accomplish if your fitness came first?

Today, I'm going to challenge you to spend the next month putting fitness first.

That's right, you get to be as selfish as you need to be in order to accomplish three goals:

You do NOT miss a workout. No matter what.

You consume healthy calories that allow you to reach your goal.

You can say no to any obligation that would keep you from getting enough sleep or working out.

When you are trying to build healthy habits, especially if you are going all in, it's often quite difficult to give yourself permission to "be selfish" when society and your duties tell you "fitness isn't a priority."

Can you put fitness first for the month and see what happens?

Physical activity – For me, it was heavy strength training and bodyweight work. But I didn't miss workouts, even when I traveled.

Nutrition – Fuel your body properly, as it's 80-90% of the battle. Get enough protein, carbs, and fats for the results YOU are looking for.

Sleep – Stop making excuses, turn off the TV, close the laptop, and get to bed on time!

We all say "I'd love to exercise more," but the reality is this: It's not what we say that is a priority, but rather what we DO that's the real priority. This is me giving you permission to give yourself permission to be selfish for a month while you're getting the ball rolling. Because it's going to be a challenge to bust through bad habits and societal pressures, this might be what you need to finally build that habit.

NOTE:

MJ West Solutions LLC Co-Founder James Ronald West is a former U.S. Soldier with over 20 years of physical trainer experience. Moreover, he is a Certified Master Personal Trainer.

REFERENCES

https://food.ndtv.com/weight-loss/these-7-fruits-can-help-you-lose-weight-1340094

http://www.omega-9oils.com/omega-9-advantage/healthier-profile/omega-3-6-9.htm

http://www.care2.com/greenliving/6-simple-recipes-for-celebrating-national-macadamia-nut-day.html

http://www.care2.com/greenliving/30-uses-for-coconut-oil.html

http://www.sustainablebabysteps.com/coconut-oil-for-weight-loss.html

http://www.care2.com/greenliving/16-health-benefits-of-lemons.html

http://www.care2.com/greenliving/15-ways-to-boost-your-liver-for-great-health.html

http://www.care2.com/greenliving/grapefruit-not-just-for-weight-loss-anymore.html

http://www.ncbi.nlm.nih.gov/pubmed/18617377

http://www.care2.com/greenliving/the-nutrient-that-burns-fat-and-boosts-energy.html

http://www.care2.com/greenliving/the-nutrient-that-burns-fat-and-boosts-energy.html

http://www.eatthis.com/weight-loss

https://naturalon.com/top-10-powerful-benefits-of-peppermint/

Additional Item Sold by MJ West Solutions

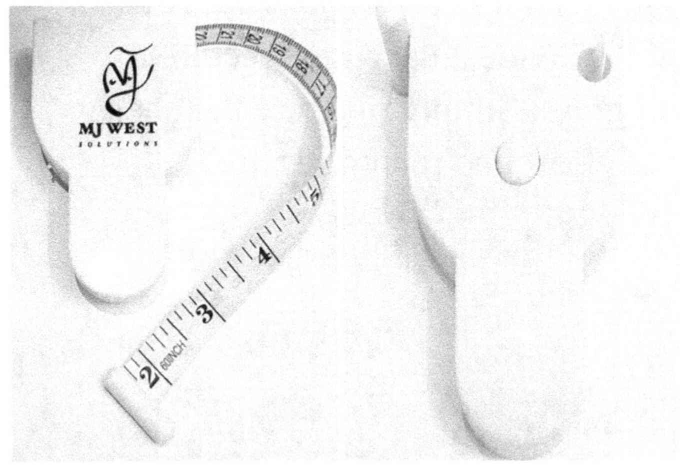

Ditch the <u>Scale</u> for the <u>Tape</u>!

Studies show scales are an inaccurate measure of progress. The average person will gain approximately one pound after consuming 16 ounces of water. As a result, their trusty scale will indicate weight gain and lack of progress. On the other hand, loss of water or lots of sweating will cause the scale to indicate weight loss and a false sense of progress. **STOP** riding on this emotional roller coaster and get on board with a true measure of progress. The MJ West Solutions Tape Measure will provide an accurate picture of progress. Simply measure the chosen body part and record results.

www.ingramcontent.com/pod-product-compliance
Lightning Source LLC
Chambersburg PA
CBHW070223260726
48658CB00006BA/2141